MIKE SPINO'S
MIND/BODY
RUNNING
PROGRAMS

MIKE SPINO

authorHOUSE®

AuthorHouse™
1663 Liberty Drive
Bloomington, IN 47403
www.authorhouse.com
Phone: 833-262-8899

Published by AuthorHouse 01/13/2023

ISBN: 978-1-6655-7991-9 (sc)
ISBN: 978-1-6655-7990-2 (e)

Edited by: Haylie Kramer

Print information available on the last page.

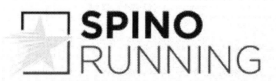

INTRODUCTION TO MIKE SPINO'S MIND/BODY RUNNING PROGRAM

I'm Coach Mike Spino, Ph.D. and I have had the privilege of training under the finest running coaches in the history of middle distance running. I have also melded it together with the most complimentary methodologies of the human potential movement of which I am a pioneer. You can find this information in my website called spinorunning.com. The training you receive on the site has been gathered from my 50 years of coaching and what I have learned about mental focusing during my years as a teacher and Director of the Esalen Sports Center within the world famous Esalen Institute

Look at my website spinorunning.com. to fill in any segments of this book, although with this book you can utilize the who website

I have put these trainings together in my website called spinorunning.com, and they have been time tested over decades and have proven extremely affective for all who utilize it. You will find your perfectly matched workouts from the three programs that are presented under the categories of emerging, initiate, and gold standard the program is for 12 weeks and goes through the segments to peak functioning and finishes with a few weeks in late May and early June when the runner is doing speed work and racing and persuadably reaching their best times of the year. In this blog for sports edtv, I will explain the reasons behind the plans being represented and how they integrate your physical running workouts, and mental training for focusing and imagination. These detailed workouts and mental training techniques go through progressive phases of from conditioning to multi-interval and classic interval training to speed workouts that allow one to reach peak functioning during the championship races of the season that matter most.

Some of these ideas are presented in my six books including *Beyond Jogging: The innerspaces of running* which can be purchased from Amazon, and has been published in numerous languages, the latest in Japanese coming out for the Christmas season. This ed tv blog contains information on ordering your program and a few videos of the mental training that is organized in what we call periodic sequences, which means matching the running the running cycle with the mental trainings so you peak, mentally and physically at the right time.

Let me explain some of the elements within the elite middle-distance running schedule you will receive by purchasing your program on spinorunning.com. A most significant contributor to my way of running training is a Hungarian born master coach Mihaly Igloi from the nation of Hungry. He emigrated to the United States after escaping the Soviet takeover of his country in 1955. At that point he had coached numerous world record holders with his method that derived from research done by the legendary scientist Gerscher and Rendell before the Second World War. The method is derived from the Freiberg interval system they developed. Basically, the running training is short intervals in sets with varying rest periods and allowing for a whole team to train together with the fastest able to at least do some training with all the others. The pair of researchers noticed that short intervals at various speeds improved middle distance times, and a number of his runners broke all world records from the 800 to 10,000 meters, on occasions that Igloi predicted.

Intervals Avoids this disturbing situation

We all know that if your group runs together for a distance run, it will break up into various sections—fast ones in the front and others behind. With an interval training everyone is able to run at least some of the workout with their mates. I have seen Igloi train four or five groups at the same time mixing and matching them and finishing their workouts at the same time. This adds to community and everyone is helping or participating with each other.

I have been coaching running and other facets of mental training for over 50 years. What if I could tell you, if you and your friends can use running as a fitness tool to be more efficiently fit, and increase your enjoyment insights. If so, I am looking for you to join in our always succeeding program. A special emphasis is placed upon the recreational program as it is the most researched and has proven the most effective.

With spinorunning.com this can happen to you! BECOME YOUR GREATEST SELF!

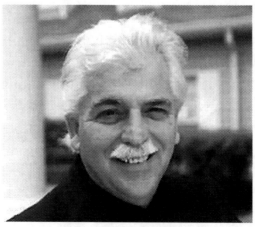

Go to Spinorunning.com to transform your LIFE.

Over the years, I keep wondering about why many aspects of running training never change. Specifically, how people incorrectly run attempting to improve fitness as well as don't use mental training in their running experiences.

Point in fact, I was teaching a workshop a few weeks ago, we were meditating with access to viewing the runners pass along a trail nearby. After we had accomplished numerous interval trainings and mental techniques, there wasn't anyone, especially changing their strides, to boost their fitness and utilize the exercise heart range (220-age and 65 to 85% percent of that number) during which we could not get into their heads there was nothing to show their inner mind was adding to the experience with Soft Eyes™ or other mind-intense techniques. It was quite astonishing actually. While Peloton and others build in the interval principle into their trainings method it does not appear to be picked up by the majority of runners in their training. If you follow the outline of the programs instilled in this program, and choose ones that match your objectives and desires you will achieve success and reach your goals.

I have written six books about mind/body running and sports viewpoints; that have been quite successful. My book, *Beyond Jogging: The innerspaces of running* has gone through numerous editions and publications and been translated into Spanish, German and Japanese. Therefore, I have embarked on this book with the publisher Author House to add to and illuminate my philosophy and techniques, and to show you how you can maximize your program in conjunction with my website spinorunning.com.

WHAT THIS BOOK WILL TEACH YOU AND YOUR FRIENDS, WHO MAY LIKE TO JOIN YOU IS A GURANTEED IMPROVEMENT IN YOUR RUNNING

There is, like for everyone, periods of growth and consolidation in one's life. You can see from the pictures in this book some of the epochs of group and individual trainings I have achieved with ongoing groups at Esalen Institute and my teams at Georgia Tech and Life University. In each, I learned, added on, and saw improvements in the fitness of my students, and better utilization of my own running mental training. Five hundred students over 14 years took my class, and used the recreational running program and had great success. Most improved between 20-25% in time and reported excellent mental training experiences. My Ph.D. is about distraction visualization, and pre-race event rehearsal. With this book you have the full training program; however, if you purchase access to the website, spinorunning.com, you will have all the accoutrements and videos that fully explain the techniques. With this book and the website, you will have a full training program especially for recreational running and cross-country and elite middle-distance running, and you also get personal mind/body running from 20 people from your corporation.

HOW I INSPIRE YOU!

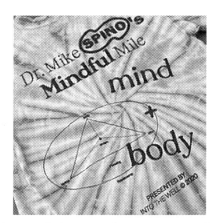

Tee shirt given to LA group in 2020 at seminar by "into the well" during a full day workshop."

There is a thin line between harping on someone to achieve something and motivating / inspiring them. Often motivational/inspirational inspirations can occur within a group of like-minded individual runners. Even within your town or community you could form a group and develop a workout plan individually and by intermingling among the group.

How to use this book in conjunction with the website.

EVERYTHING YOU NEED IS IN THIS BOOK AND YOU CAN view the WEBSITE (spinorunning.com) if purchased separately.

The objective of Mike Spino's Mind/Body Running Program book is to learn more efficient, more insightful running. It is created in unison with spinorunning. com website. However, together, you will have a step-by-step plan, and you will be able to use it in conjunction with the website and be more observant.

- First, the Spino mind/body running program is individualized, in both the one mile program for beginners and adaptions of the 5k for more seasoned runners. I like to start people at the mile, and there is an adaption for the treadmill that I instituted during the Covid epidemic.

- The mental training is within the program (like Soft Eyes™ and Wipe Away™) and part of the techniques that blend into your run. They are all designed to make fitness easier to attain and more enjoyable to experience.

- The recreational program has been proven in research by 500 college students who improved at least 20% and reported positive reactions over the mental training components

- The phases represented in the elite middle-distance running has produced many personal results and numerous 4-minute milers.

- The cross-country program depicted has created many national champions.

- You can see recent interviews my youtube channel at https://youtube.com/@spinnorunning

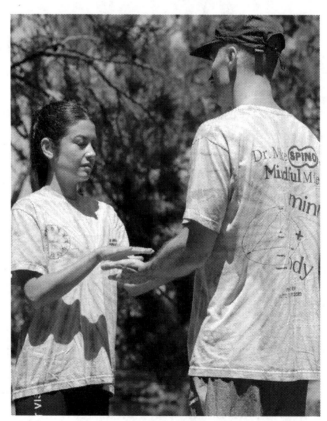

Setting up energy transfer for duo training

LEARN EVERYTHING ABOUT BREATHING FIRST, THE REST WILL FOLLOW

<u>To Start we first breathe and think!</u>

Breathing is thought of as a natural, unconscious process; however, in running, it is more diverse than what may first be imagined. Sagas have been asked the question what they would do when real tragedy or exultation occurred, and they would say "simply breathe." The supposition is that if you can pause and breathe, you have the ability to put the present into focus more easily. It is a basic component and registers with everything that happens with you whether you are stationary or when breathing.

Numerous ideas have come forth about breathing while running, the Finns were thought to have some secrets such as inhaling on particular steps; however, there method eventually became unstable when the speed intensified. My belief is much simpler: it is at every opportunity exhale imperceptivity and wait for the lungs to fill up, by raising your shoulders and being observant of what your body does naturally. There are numerous exercises on the website and in my books about recovery and most of them are about raising your shoulders and waiting that is preceded by first exhaling.

Most runners think that when you run you get out of breath, and then are forced to slow down or stop. Breathing is more volitional, and there are many dimensions in the way it can function. First, the exhale is the key factor and is more impactful on breathing than the inhale.

Try this little experiment to reveal how and why this is so. Start by standing stationary and exhaling from the belly area of your body. Then wait, and when next you inhale, raise your shoulders for full aeration and recognize the entire capacity of your lungs.

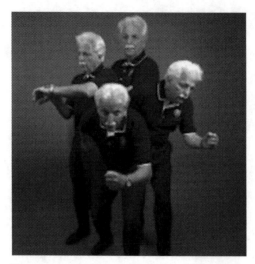

Various phases of timing of coaching

This little breathing exercise provides a little introduction to the diversity for breath, and a first step into the amazing functions of breathing while running. The problem for most runners is that they have little awareness of how their lungs, the powerhouse within one's running physiology, are working, and therefore have no tools to ward off fatigue when it is occurring. The techniques that follow will add a lot to your breathing capacity while running.

My coach, the legendary Percy Wells Cerutty of Australia, concentrated on breathing as a tool for increasing endurance. See "Tidal Breathing" in the Recreational in the Recreational section of the website to see how tidal breathing functions to replenish and refresh.

BREATHING: THE TIDAL BREATH™

Breathing can be thought of as a series of ocean waves. Watch them and gain knowledge from nature. They come to shore with different forces and velocities; no two are the same.

The ebb and flow of the tides, each unique, and in constant change, teach us about the comparability of life in all its moods and potentialities.

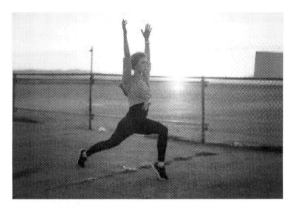

Breathing at a District Vision seminar

Watch the "Recreational" section of my website and you will see both a Cerutty athlete practicing the technique and then a woman (actually my daughter) doing a tidal breath.

Tidal breathing is also enormously effective for beginning (recreational) runners. The picture below is my class doing a tidal breath is instructional. Below is the best photograph of a tidal breath in action taken by Chadwick Tyler, who gave me the District Vision Name "Captain Mike." His unique vision and insight captured a perfect example of the tidal breath, and my dear friend, Max Vallot, pictured on the right is doing it perfectly, as are the others in the photo.

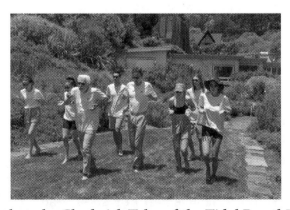

Amazing photo by Chadwick Tyler of the Tidal Breath™ in action

Tidal breathing is applied during an interval, about halfway into the interval, at what we call the acceleration point. To gain from it while running, first, exhale, and then take a breath in unison with your arms coming up your sides to a point at the top of your diaphragm; then hold it for a split second, and turn your hands towards the ground thereby allowing yourself to thrust forward.

It is important to keep the arms close to your sides (like in the photograph) and coming up like an elevator and then release the breath and thrust forward. Your heart range will be increased as you expel your breathe. The movement should be streamlined and not make forward movement more cumbersome or hold you back from the acceleration. So, arms are close to your sides, exhaling and raising your shoulders getting maximum breath to propel forward.

Additionally, when running along in a race, the tendency when tiring is to gasp for breath, however, this impends rather than assists. It is better to exhale and place your awareness below your navel and wait for the inevitable inhale to replenish your lungs. When doing this let the breath come naturally into your abdomen, rise into your diaphragm and then chest, and 'sigh' thereby warding off the anaerobic debt.

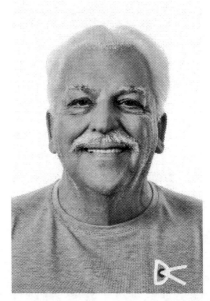

Buy my course at districtvision.com for $9, and you get a lot of information and receive clarity about the techniques covered.

Remember, it is not a linear passage to the anaerobic threshold where lactic acid presumably slows forward motion. Consciousness and breathing techniques, can ward off fatigue. Too many runners believe running should be a silent endeavor without much sound and at a constant tempo until tired.

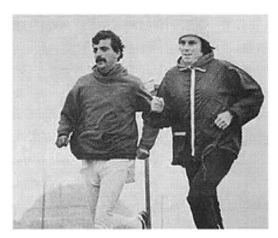

Running with Esalen Founder Michael Murphy in 1974

The opposite is true. Another fun technique that increases the exercise heart range in workshops, and always makes the group laugh together, is called the Surge™ and is done by making a sound (like Bing) in the epiglottis while surging forward, thereby increasing the heartbeat into the upper part of the exercise heart range.

When having to double in a meet or running at high altitude: Also, a breathing exercise to do before a race or hard practice that helps those with exercise asthma is called breathing coordination. During the 1968 Olympics in Mexico City, distance runners were worried about the high altitude of 6,800 feet. Should one come early to acclimate or right before the meet and hope the altitude doesn't have a major effect?

This was a challenge Dr. Carl Strough faced with his experiments with the Yale track team. Again, lactic acid is not a straight line. When it comes, it is debilitating, and it reaches a point at which you are unable to run, but it can be backed off from and regulated quite successfully.

What Dr. Strough (aka Dr. Breath) deemed a simple exercise, is to increase the number of counts you can have with an exhale.

Here is how it works: Breathing Coordination

Let all the air out of your lungs, while at a prone position on the floor, and fill your lungs up counting out loud. It is easy to hit 30 or 40 numerically (you are exhaling while you breathe), and then, slightly force the rest of the breath out. After that is accomplished, fill up your lungs in increments of 10 and exhale letting the rest of the air out. Usually at about a number between 60 or as much as 80 no more breath can be expelled. I have found this an effective technique to do especially between races if one is doubling in two events. It relaxes the lungs and has them "practice" breathing and gets one's lungs ready, much as a singer finds the place in his or her breath from which to hit any high pitches.

Remember, breathing is most recuperative when starting from the belly. Some coaches talk about surface breathing to quickly get air into the lungs for a quick renewal. It is helpful in some situations, although my practice with runners is to help them determine how they can empty their lungs, to make the inhale more recuperative. I teach this as a recovery, abet, it is called Standing Breathing Recovery, and I have videos on my websites to see how it is accomplished.

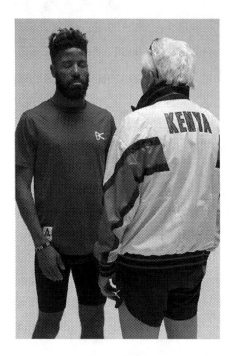

The fantastic thing with intervals is that it is beneficial to stop and start again with rest periods that allow for particular and planned recoveries. I recommend runners do a Standing Breath Recovery amidst a run with maybe a few segments, like doing three sets of 10-minute intervals. The runner can combine this method with what I call the Full Body Recovery which is recommended after the workout is complete to check the body for tightness and/or potential injuries. These two methods can be done together by utilizing visualized color while tightening and relaxing the muscles and ligaments of the body.

Focus areas can be done in these exercises also by tightening and relaxing parts of your body. On the release let the body part or area relax. For instance, like "scrunching" the feet and imagining colors into areas that might be tight or slightly painful. Follow throughout the body like bending one's knees and straightening and concentrating breath and color into the hamstrings and then the abdomen, chest, and upper diaphragm.

Finding areas of your body to concentrate upon is also helpful when one wants to concentrate their energy in the middle of the body, shortened stride (this help you from stepping out too long). Place the finish line. You will in your mind and imagine being pulled towards it; even employ Soft Eyes™ to imagine being pulled towards the finish. You see running is not just arms and thighs; it is the whole body and especially what is happening in your mind's eye as you shift mentally and physically (as you do naturally) in your mind's eye.

For instance, holding your face in a warrior's sensibility can be done by concentrating just below the eyes and letting one's countenance be strong and fearless. As you are now seeing, running is not one-dimensional; a lot more is happening.

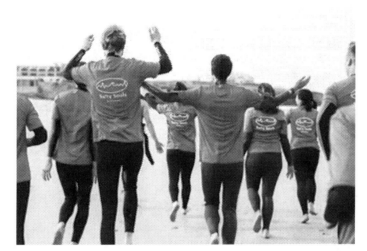

Corporate training can change your whole company for the better
Spino Running Shorts by District Vision (DistrictVision.com)

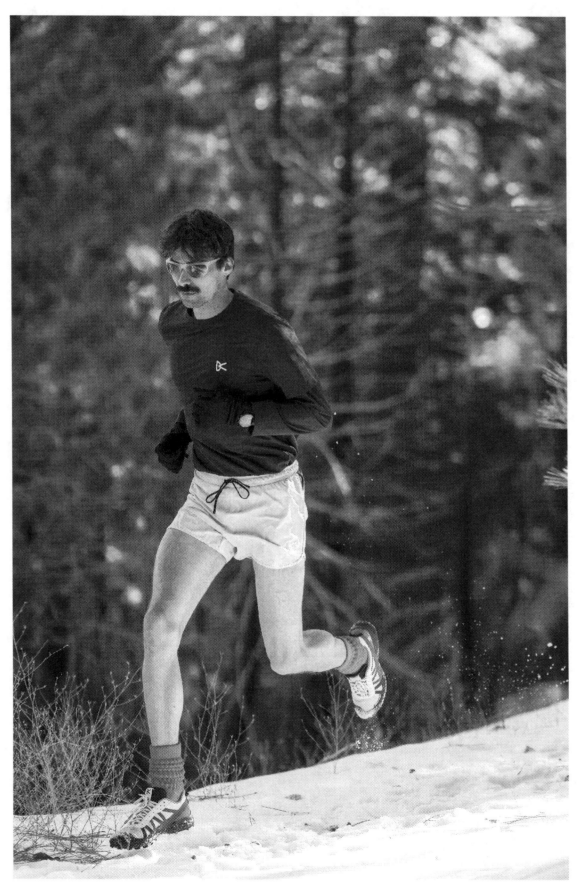

In conclusion, now you see there are numerous mental frameworks. The mind is one of the most diverse aspects of the running body. Understanding your mind/body connection is one of the keys to integrating your running. Doing mind/body running exercises melds yourself together. I recommend forms of periodic training to sequence together phases of training. There is an overlap when one goes from one period of training to the other. It will feel uncomfortable at first until the sequence is blended into the new form of training. As you begin with full-body recovery, and basic relaxation exercises, you will get closer to knowing what your mind is doing as it slows down.

You are now ready to utilize more complex mental training such as guided imageries in event rehearsals in practice and just before a race. The semblance of unity the runner seeks in his or her practice is a combination of proper interval training from conditioning to speed and racing, as well as pinpointing the mental training that matches the training cycles you are accomplishing. I hope this chapter has given some insight into the functions that are optimum for peak experiences.

This book supplements my website spinorunning.com. From the website you can get a better understanding about numerous techniques like gaits and tempos. You will also find voice instruction and videos on items like meditation and relaxation, as well as an excellent rendition of my 24 step method demonstrated by my nephew, Derek Verde.

WHAT GUIDED IMAGERY CAN ADD TO YOUR PERFORMANCE

We start with the mind's connection to the body to begin

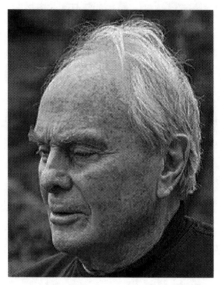

Michael Murphy meditating

Guided Imagery adds power to your action

If you have the proper imagery in your mind, it can be a big benefit to sport action. Following is instruction on guided imagery, sometimes called visualization. If done properly, this technique can really get a runner out of his or her head and emotions and lead to more focused and direct reality. Let's look at how great athletes accomplish this focusing, and how they get into a mental framework that allows them to accomplish successful feats.

HOW DO ATHLETES VISUALIZE SUCCESS AND HOW IT IS ACCOMPLISHED?

The great football player, Jim Brown, from my school, Syracuse University, could do amazing things on the football field like cutting for the correct hole and thrusting himself into the open field. Spectators saw this while on the field; however, they didn't witness the mental planning he did within the locker room or how he was led by a sport psychologist or mental trainer beforehand. Every kid does a visualization in his home net when he says, "3,2,1" and swishes a basketball. I did it with my childhood friends; it is the essence of being a hero to the home crowd.

Mental imagery is enhanced by practice. Guided imagery is when there are gaps in the narrative with the intension of the athlete filling in the blanks with his/her best scenario. Visualization is following a line guide to the end of a narrative that comes out ideally. Imagery can be internal or external, seeing yourself from outside going towards, say, a camera. Internal is feeling from within yourself and external viewing from outside. One has to be careful during the visualization as research shows some processes don't work well for particular people. For instance, research on a high school cross-country team reveals that internal visualization can make female cross-country runners uncomfortable, while external is a little easier for them to experience.

<u>The first element is learning to relax yourself than mind/body is easier to explore.</u>

When your mind/body is scattered, it isn't easy to do visualizations or guided imagery. That is why it is preferable to practice meditation first a few times a week before apply guided imagery or visualization.

Then, afterwards, your mind is more open to mind/body suggestions. People do visualization or guided imagery the first time after practicing basic meditation for a few weeks. The "jumpy mind" isn't ready for visualization or guided imagery without learning to calm yourself. You need to work on calming your mind first and foremost. In the interview section portion of the website, there is a interview I did with Ian Dube on basic meditation and another with Donna Garcia within recreational running.

Because meditation is so essential, it is presented in various parts of the website. The most basic practice for relaxation meditation is to begin breathing as you count, "one" on the inhale and "two" on the exhale. My friend, Max Vallot, at District Vision (<u>www.districtvision.com</u>) teaches by pausing for a split second on the inhale, as well as on the exhale. Count one on each inhale, pause, and then two on the exhale, and so forth. As you practice this breathing by counting to four each time, you probably will lose your count occasionally. That is alright; just return to one and start again.

Once the breathing smooths out and you can count through to four quite easily, it is time to cease the counting and let your mind give way to your thoughts randomly. Let them simply roll through your mind. If you feel you have been having a little trouble, go back to counting to four again, monitoring your thinking. At this point, after about four weeks doing this for 10 minutes per day or so, it is time to begin visualization and guided imagery because, by this time, you can carry an image into a sport or game and effectively calm your mind\ body getting ready for the imagery. We call this the induction.

After perhaps a few weeks of this simplified meditation, you are ready to do a lead in to your visualization or guided imagery. This is begun with a technique called *centering*. Centering develops your ability to develop composure in action. When centering succeeds for an individual, he/she can adjust unconsciously to the psycho-physical demands of the game. In other words, the mental and physical alignments that must be continually evaluated in a game can occur unconsciously.

These are videos and explanations you will find on the website

Videos: Donna and Mike (end of recreational running)

- * **tidal breathing**
- * **surging**
- * **relax and concentration**
- * **energy transfer**
- * **audio interview with Ian Dube**

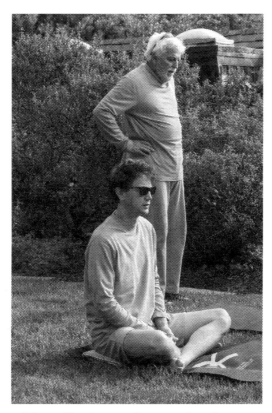

Max Vallot and I meditating and preparing for a running session

Being centered means that your movements are directed towards a specific goal without being distracted. Physically, this springs from the area in your belly. Centering allows your movements to be coordinated and occur automatically.

Technique: Begin by standing face to face with someone. One person begins to walk forward while the other person places his hand on his partner's chest and offers resistance. The person walking against the hand will notice that when his breath awareness is located at the center of his body, (known to the Chinese as "tandem"), it is easier to move against the resisting hand. Repeat for three or four time for about 40 meters each time, alternating sides with partners so that each partner gets a kinesthetic sense of being centered.

WHAT CAN WE LEARN BY WATCHING OLYMPIANS?

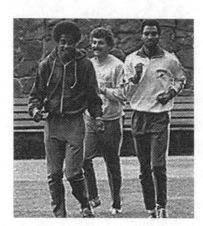

Running with the Guys of Pro Track-1974

We watch Olympians execute beautifully, as they move effortlessly, smoothly, and in control. What appears as automatic fluidity is, however, a combination of muscle memory from hard work and repetition, as well as applied mental energy.

The internal balance and composure that they display is what the non-elite athlete among us wants to attain, isn't it? How can we, as recreational athletes, have the same experiences as Olympians? We can't fully; however, I have a supposition that, to a certain extent, we all can. It takes a self-release from convention and an understanding beyond ordinary channels, as well as a commitment to a mind/body method of operating. It also requires a look at what is not so wonderful about high-level completion and the demise it may cause to a competitive athlete's long-term mental health.

Successful, professional coaches should know that insulting athletes only diminish themselves, and their athlete and is not in the spirit of sportsmanship expected. Outstanding coaches get the most elegant and fluid performances from their athletes by understanding them in a personalized manner. Some people may think well of "tough-minded" coaches pounding the training into their charges by goading and intimidation. This has a very limited effectiveness, perhaps when teaching basic drills; however, insightful, effective coaches see and sense success beyond these limited perspectives.

The recreational athlete might struggle with their own clarity, and usually does not have the feedback of professional coaches; however, we can self-plan and be rewarded with similar mind/body outcomes. While recreational athletes do not have as highly talented coaches as Olympians and do have their limitations, there is a path ahead, and it can be established by small, nuanced techniques that are integrative for the mind and body. Some examples may be expository as we see in high level mental trainers. As far back as the 1960s, sports psychologists like Lars Eric Unesthal of Sweden observed the actions of top-level athletes and categorized them. He noted that Wayne Gretsky knew where the puck was going before it got there. He has researched the proven effectiveness of mental training for over 60 years. Another good friend, NFL linebacker David Meggyessy, had many a premonitions as to where the next play would go. He would go to that spot to make magnificent tackles.

Furthermore, how do the great coaches like my mentor Percy Wells Cerutty of Australia know exactly how to motivate particular athletes, like World Record Holder and Gold Medalist Herb Elliott, and have the secrets of how to motivate human behavior. Perceptive coaches know motivation is not the same for everyone. I once had a trio of Olympic-level runners that were differently by their internal sensibilities. One wanted to hear the "Star Spangled Banner," another had impressions about the starting line and existentialism, and the third was dealing with negative thoughts he had built up over time. During the football season, it was said that NFL coach Vince Lombardi drove his family crazy with his temperament but had a keen perspective as to what buttons to press to get the most out of his players.

Such is the talk about the crème de la crème of athletes where there is beauty to behold. A local football referee in awe of the abilities of Peyton Manning in high school was distracted while noticing how proficient he was and couldn't believe a high school kid could be so amazing. The example of gymnast Simone Biles' mental preparation that at once sky-rocketed her to the top and brought her to her knees is instructional. However, while these sterling performers are a thrill to behold, it doesn't have that much to do with possibly the worldwide struggle of the modern person to find some grace and elegance in a world full of Covid, Cancer, and every kind of illness supposedly cured by pills and injections. How does the everyday athlete discover a semblance of harmony and elegant action that transcends their ordinary concerns?

The secret is to begin with small steps towards your goals. This can be accomplished through mental and breathing techniques such as what's known as Progressive Relaxation (PR). PR was created and named by internist, psychologist, and physiologist Edmund Jacobsen. He noticed that if one breathes while tightening and relaxing individual muscle groups of the body, calmness will be achieved. Through these types of small steps, even as small as 30 to 40 seconds of looking inward, the mind/body process is put into effect. This can be aided by the Soft Eyes™.

This means recognizing elements within yourself by looking inward and outward at the same time. If you see an Olympian closing their eyes just before they begin a movement, you can bet they are visualizing the steps of their upcoming technique. It is not so much that this will end up exactly as planned and Olympians may have to improvise as they go along, but it is a big step in the right direction. Gold medalist swimmer, Mark Spitz, even visualized out-swimming sharks as an intense motivation; whereas, Michael Phelps increased his mental focus to just squeeze out races for the gold medals.

The all-time NFL running back, Jim Brown, would visualize plays and optional "holes" in the defense. He was so good at it that when he approached the line of scrimmage, he could veer in any direction naturally. The athlete needs to transition to the melding of mind and body to experience something different about one's self.

The aspects become clearer and the person changes almost imperceptibly but they sense it as do their compatriots, coaches and friends. That's how mind/body changes appear for all people. When accomplished; it is observable to the talented eye. As a track coach, I have a concept of "carry" when someone is improving. The tasks somehow are easier and the "reserve power" begins to appear to oneself. Mind/body is less perceptible to observers; however, it is more than real to the person experiencing it. It is the new, whole you.

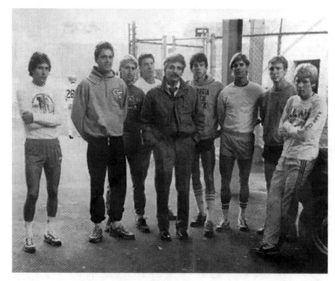

My team at Georgia Tech including four who were four-minute milers

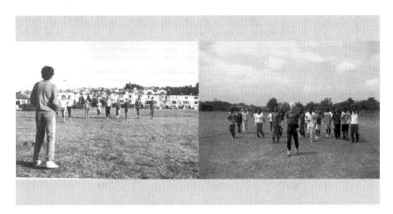

Share This Story, Choose Your Platform!

On Website spinorunning.com: See Donna and Coach Spino meditating, hear Video of Relaxation Audio by Ian Dube interview

<u>Do this short memory image a few moments before the critical part of the game.</u>

All: You are now facing the climax of the game or event. There is still a feeling of kinesthetic grace and ideal form as you are waiting for the perfect moment at which to release your final reserves of speed and power. When you are secure, knowing that when you give the signal, your body will respond instantly.

<u>Here is an example in your running</u>

Runner: Now you are making your final thrust, opening your throttle. When you do, the energy and power you expected comes forth in full measure. As you approach and pass others, your energy and determination double and each new talent is like the first. As you cross the finish line, you feel intensely aware of your own courage and determination. Looking at the clock you notice you have run the time you set for yourself. You are happy and satisfied with your achievement.

THE ATHLETE OF THE FUTURE

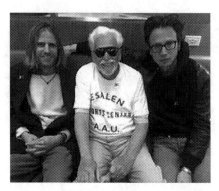

The wonderful Tom Daly and Max Vallot founders of District Vision

My training shorts can be found under apparel in the DistrictVision.com website

Almost 50 years ago in my book, *Beyond Jogging: the inner spaces of running.* I wrote a chapter entitled, "The Athlete of The Future." What I have discovered in the time since, is that some things have are changed in perspective; others have already come true; some are now recognized realities. This short article. which appeared in sportsedtv provides insights for the impending potentials which probably certainly become part of our daily sport experience. Some might be in evolution and difficult to recognize where they will eventually settle. Of course, in sports and overall life we have lived a half century since this chapter was first written; championship athletes are probably better than ever, and the mental training practice is more abundant.

In the 1970s sport had not yet been tarnished with dope scandals, and the likes of Lance Armstrong, Ben Johnson, Barry Bonds and Marion Jones had not been front-page news. Drugs being tossed into the mix contributes to the blurred lines of my viewpoint; because now, it is a cat and mouse game as athletes are masking their drug use to mask their utilization. Only now during the world events like the Olympics do we hear about drugs, although the entire Russian Federation for Track and Field has been banned from the Olympics. However, we don't hear about illegal drugs too often anymore. Maybe it's being masked better.

Get your corporation involved—I will get everyone fit and happy
https://districtvision.com/products/spino-5-training-shorts-black

The Amble from Percy Cerutty

Sport performance is continually explored, then for other goals, that were in many ways more alarming. With drugs there was the realization of being able to train hard with less fatigue but had many side effects like hostility to others and long-term dangers such as brain cancer. In a recent study, athletes were asked if they would give up five years of their lives to win an Olympic medal, and many said they would be happy to.

I prefer to know the self and its ups and downs rather than to have performance enhanced. The true self might be hard to accept, but it is truthful. The language of sport has only slightly evolved, since drugs became a part of the story, and the foresight of my good friends, Michael Murphy and his human performance colleagues are continually searching and finding new sources of inspiration.

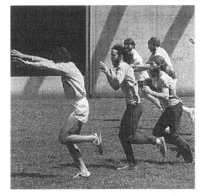

The Amble I learned from Percy Cerutty as the second step (after the stretch up) in learning to *gallop*.

I will attempt to follow some main points *of Beyond Jogging*, although the vantages at present might be skewered in new directions. For instance, the athlete of the future will still be using a whole new array of methods, orientations and approaches to sport and concentrate on a fresh sense of the mind. These frontiers will always be exponentials, as many more mental strategies reaching clear mentality will be discovered and probed for effectiveness. Calling on all the research as far back as the East German's hidden potentials programs and expansive human potentials techniques, athletes, and especially recreational athletes, will have little use for performance enhancements and obtain better insights into themselves. I know and sense this as fact of explorations in every direction seem to point this out.

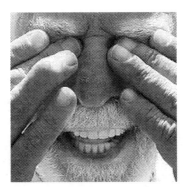

**The Wipe Away™ technique—use this after a moving
visualization (like Soft Eyes™) to return to present realities.**

There will be a new sense that we bring our entire self into the game, and it will be recognized as a reflection of our fuller selves. Athletic people in the future will be concerned with coordinating physical and psychic experiences. In this context, a new language will emerge which better describes various situations, from feeling smooth and coordinated to clearer; awareness and actual clumsiness at every level will be improved upon. Athletic journalists, will attempt to describe the extraordinary, like Steph Curry's long one hander. This will come to fore through mind/body interactives. Athletes will be transformed from being reticent about explorations to an eagerness to explore. This is my prophecy.

This happened to me in my first mystical experience. I wrote about it in the story, "Running as a Spiritual Experience." It made me want more, and it came, but in new and unexpected ways that set me up to write my first poetry book because now I saw and could recall the mental gymnastics at play. Like the outer space lingo that was adopted after Sputnik. Concepts such as timelessness, precognition and space/time lapse became valid ingredients of sport and continue to be ones we all will seek, cherish and converse about with similar people who are luckily affected.

An athlete of the future, a runner, for instance, will pay attention to the perambulation of style as well as the speed and the distances that are covered. Practices like Rolfing, chiropractic manipulation and all types of body rearrangement like Feldenkrais' exercises (his book is called *Awareness Through Movement)* will help all move with new efficiency and continue to be ones we all will seek.

The Wipe Away™ technique for clearing an image

Eastern and Western philosophies will meet in a blending of disciplines, and the great athletes will be recognized as heroes of the spirit. In this context, all athletes will demand a larger utilization of the self and ways to receive it. The auras and the energy fields, the human biofield around our bodies, will be recognized, as athletes may perform rituals of centering and visualizations before sport activity. These practices will integrate into all aspects of the self— intuition, sensing, thinking and feeling into sport. In this framework athletics will become a source of self-knowledge. Soon, after the taping for Saturday's football game is complete, you may hear hour-long sessions in which music, exercise, and suggestions will be made to the team, so that they emerge from the locker room with increased awareness, sometimes even in a trance that careful observers will be able to recognize.

There will be an attempt to modernize approaches and methods, but will still also be the realization that the roots of athletics go deep, and while it is important to improve, it is important also not to lose a sense of tradition. Natural rather than prefabricated principles will appear from closer observation of natural states; children will learn to walk differently, so they may be as quick as kittens and gallop like horses. There will be a reemphasis on relaxation. Methods such as Feldenkrais' exercises that break up fixed patterns of mind and body will make a body more sensitive and able to transform this new body reality into various movement formats. When movements are practiced in relaxed ways, we will recognize resistors to fluid motion. The mind and all the ramifications of inner space will be incorporated in the body's achievements. The truth found in stillness will be transferred to the athletic act. Instances like Arthur Ashe meditating between sets at Wimbledon visualizing events and dreaming plans will play sports a challenge of the mind's as well as bodies.

The athlete will train in part like a dancer, stretching each ligament and joint to maximum strength. Within it all, there will be a sense of changed realities that are carried along, sometimes enperceptively. The athlete will strengthen the body with barbells and other devices and elastic rubber, so that all the parts are more flexible and mobile. There will be a better understanding of anatomy, and the ways and means of body movement. This will create a new way of body action. There will be a new training method which incorporates musculoskeletal exercises, inner space awareness and more precise kinesthetic sensations. These new disciplines will make available extraordinary realities not before accessible through training preparation. The places entered by these voyages may seem dangerous, and there will be the understanding that true adventure often means the courage for free fall.

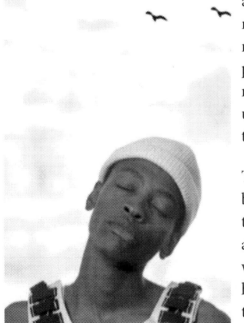

How to set up Soft Eyes™ by visualizing birds in the trees

There should be no sanctity about the new way but simply the realization that athletics has been taught in a metaphorical Ice Age, and that we seek a renaissance. The knowledge of previous teachers will be important, myself included, so that not to have to relieve the same steps again and go over the same pathways and have to learn it all again. My teachers, Percy Cerutty and Michael Murphy, taught me to be aware, not try to have the same experience twice and to be courageous. Like an

Irish runner who never ran in a race but did run a mile under 4:10 and soon died on the spot. The information of the past and the old renaissance will be necessary to have had coaching teams that stayed current and looked for openings for new explorations. In the future, however, it will not be uncommon for an athlete or even a weekend warrior to have a session of polarity massage, followed by an hour of guided fantasy, and a session of Feldenkrais' exercises before and after a game, so he or she can rebalance. In conjunction with training, or during the off season, he/she may delve into structural integration, bioenergetics, join an ongoing interpersonal group or study aikido or tai chi. An athlete of every dimension can do many things, especially if the goal is inner satisfaction, and one exercise isn't exhausting, like a 15-mile run would be. Emphasis will be on preparation of the total person. Excellence in the sport or game will be a by-product.

Intercollegiate sports, college club teams, will lose their exclusively physical emphasis and will mesh with humanities and philosophy. Physical education will be taught from the inside as well as the outside. Nutrition will play an important part. We will learn not only what foods are best for health purposes, but what should be consumed in periods of extended activity, just before strenuous acts or when the body needs recovery.

It was discovered by the Russians that through a carbohydrate build up in the days before competition, performance could be maximized by eating the correct food. Athletes, like footballer Tom Brady at 45, have understood how this works and have a food regimen that allows them to still want to play and set records.

Pills and stimulants will cease to be crutches. The general consensus will be that the variance caused by these outside influences robs us of our personal resources. Finally, and not so easily said, there will be a different feeling surrounding athletic events. Yes, there will be the dark side where spectators visualize spiders in an opponent's muscles, but the wonderful sense will be presented. Like the video, "The Joy of Sox," by Dr. Rick Lefkowitz. It tells of the love of the Boston Red Sox fans that extended into winning a World Series. So many New Yorkers were fans of 1950s baseball when three teams, the Yankees, the Giants and the Dodgers graced the New York City community with ceaseless admiration.

Individuals who have prepared for an event will see it as their day to shine and experience their special day together with other competitors. The training preparation and build-up will be seen as a preparation rite for the voyage into the physical/spiritual world, and we will have some sense that our bodies belong to us but may be part of a vast oneness and that each rite we enter into will take us closer to our larger potentials.

Cross-country Precedes Track for Most Distance Runners

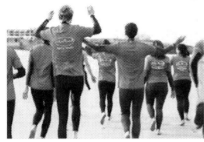

**Corporate Running—
Running together will add a
linkage to your organization!**

Cross-country training is a process that starts in the warm summer months and ends in the chill of late autumn. It is, above all else, an activity of cycles. It is a 13-16 week season during, which the coach and team are beginning with a new base of conditioning and a year ahead full of promise and ambition. This article provides instruction in the workouts, drills and methods used for each segment of the cross-country season.

The suggestions outline an ideal season of training, although we will also speak about how to handle injury and setback, so you can learn how to regroup and peak during the championship part of the season. At the end of this, a means for reviewing how to evaluate the most important elements of the training process is explained.

PLANNING THE PRE-SEASON

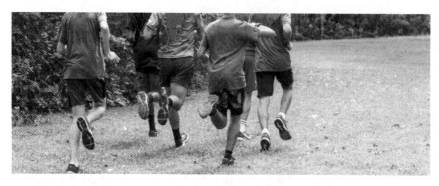

The season's initial set-up for the high school, college, university and post-collegiate coach has some dissimilarity. It is recommended that the first pre-season workouts begin on a flat grass field. We hope this minimizes a workout we call "the long sad gray line," which refers to the practice of mostly high school coaches to have their team run for an indiscriminate time along the streets with the lead runner striding smoothly in front and everyone else straggling behind. Rather from the beginning, our method emphasizes selective group training. The coach's objective is to figure out whom to train with whom, and what workouts and what sequence of workouts will get the entire team at full throttle when it counts most—during the championship part of the season. The genius of all groupers was Hungarian born Mihaly Igloi. He was coach to many star runners who used his method for vast improvement. His mastery could be observed in watching 30 to 40 runners, in six or seven groups, doing all manner of workouts in different directions and at various speeds and finishing the workout together. The successful cross-country coach does not have to be this precise; however, understanding the nuances of applying workouts that are physiologically semi accurate and diverse is at the heart of this program

SEGMENTS OF THE YEAR-LONG PROGRAM

The flat grass surface should be at least as large as the inside of a football field, and if possible, accessible to locations for long, continuous running. As in all successful periodization training, each segment has a goal, methods and techniques to achieve a particular result that naturally plateaus before it blends into the next phase of training. The coach teaches new techniques and terms in each phase of the training, and the methods are broken down into the physical and mental aspects of the workout. Each new phase of the season will have the group return to the grass field to learn additional techniques that are then integrated into the whole program. The goal is for all aspects of the training and for each runner in the group to reach the zenith of peak performance during the championship phase of the season

Pre-Season Workouts

The initial phase of training is the pre-season that, in the US, lasts from July to the end of August. In the pre-season, the goal is to learn the initial techniques that are applied in the interval part of the training plan. Our aim in all phases is to keep all team members injury-free as an aerobic base of conditioning is established. The unique training techniques are physical and mental, as the team is training physically but also learning how to utilize lung and mental capacities to their maximum potentials.

Gaits and Tempos of Running—Initial Drills for Teaching Gaits and Tempos

The pre-season begins with instruction in the application of gaits and tempos methodology. To accomplish this, the coach can face the team directly on the grass field and lead or have a team member demonstrate the forms and speeds of running used in our interval training. We all know that effective training takes a sensibility of pace and an understanding of the best forms of running movement to achieve physiological efficiency. Using perhaps a straightaway of 100 meters, the coach explains that a gait is the form of movement during the run and that the tempo is the velocity at which you move. As the coach gives these gaits and tempos names, he is developing a language to communicate his training instructions and a means to carry out his training instructions. Igloi's terminology works well in this regard as fresh swing tempo, is assuming a gait and velocity up to about 60% effort. Good swing tempo approaches speeds from 60 to 80%, and hard swing tempo is between 80-95% effort.

During the entire season, each training phase has at least one and usually two days of training on this grass field. The terminology, however, can be used on all surfaces and workouts during the entire season. One of the main reasons for using the gait and tempo with the whole group initially is to make sure each runner has time to "regroup," so the workout retains group unity. The stopwatch should be used sparingly at the beginning of the season. When used properly, the stopwatch should determine the level of conditioning rather than be a means of setting up workouts to get in shape. In the pre-season, the team learns mid-pace running, so as to maximally utilize the Exercise Heart Range (220-age and 60-85% of the target numbers) and avoid sprinting that places the runners' physiology over the anaerobic threshold where it shuts down its capacities because of the presence of lactic acid.

The three weeks of pre-season will contain two kinds of workouts—intervals and long continuous runs. Interval workouts have a particular sequence of warm-up, stretching, the body of the workout and a recovery method.

For the warm-up during pre-season, the coach can instruct with the following information:

- Warm-Up During Pre-Season: After the team jogs together for about five minutes; finish the warm-up with a few easy stretches and a technique called *the shake-up*

The following stretches are good for starters:

- *Full Body Swing:* Feet shoulder width apart, raise your arms and extend to the sides swinging your entire body from right to left.

- *Grape Picker:* Slowly stretch both hands overhead, then stretch your right hand as high as possible and repeat on the left side as if you were picking grapes.

- *Lateral Stretch:* Raise right arm straight overhead, palms up, as you place your left hand on your left hip. Bend as far as possible to the left while reaching over and down to the left with your right arm. Repeat on the other side.

- *Wall Stretch:* Leaning on a wall or tree, move your right foot back about two feet and place your heel down, toes straight. Lean into the wall bending the left foot forward and allow your right leg to stretch. Repeat on the other side.

- *Skip and Shake-Up:* On the grass field, take a distance of maybe 60 meters and begin by skipping as a child skips, only raising your knees a bit higher. Shake up by letting your muscles hang like a rag doll. Every so often, throw your hands over your head and to the sides but stay mainly on your toes to loosen up our body and elevate your heartbeat to get ready for the workout. Up and down the 60 meters about four times is usually good to complete the warm-up.

Begin the first workout by teaching the difference between fresh, good and hard swing. Have your team run at the various tempos and they will naturally assume the gait that accomplishes the objective. The coach will do perhaps three or four 100-meter intervals with a rest period between each, so the group can regather together after each segment.

Introduction of the breathing drills

Breathing Drills— Our Breath is our Awareness

The breathing techniques are taught on the grass field using the concept of the acceleration point. Usually accomplished just once at the point of acceleration, the technique known as tidal breathing propels the runner into a faster tempo half way into the interval. The coach can explain the following breathing principles to his team while standing in front of them on the grass field:

- The exhale is the starting point of all breathing techniques. The sound of the exhale should reverberate like the sound of a hollow log.

- When you use the full capacity of your lungs, your breathing begins in the diaphragm and rises to the top of your chest filling up like a balloon.

- Stored breath released properly can help accelerate you forward.

- Relaxing your lungs, when stationary, in between parts of the workout accelerates physical recovery.

This will get you started. Look at spinorunning.com for more suggestions.

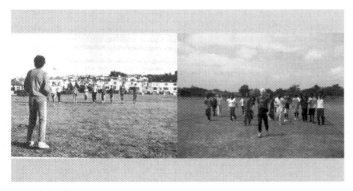

Michael Spino Michael Spino, Ph.D., is the founder and CEO of Spino Running and The Mindful Runners [...]

S.F Group and Kenyan Research Group

How to train and peak for middle-distance running

Let's look at training for distance running beginning with cross-country to the peaking during the late outdoor track season. The training is broken up into emerging, initiate and elite runners from middle school through college and beyond. It is also in track broken into conditioning, multi-intervals, classic intervals, speed sets and peaking These runners are unique boys and girls, young men and women who train year round and pinpoint each period that transitions into the next.

You will find the periods of transition satisfying. It is always difficult at first, but happy and ready for the change to the next period of training. Peaking will provide real happiness as you have come through a cycle and feel different. Many will notice that some skills like hard continuous running gets boring in the last phase of peaking and just jogging or good swing will be sufficient.

There are now millions of young people running cross-country and middle-distance races from 800 meters to 5,000 meters throughout the world. While it is a relatively easy task to put together a customary schedule of training for these events, the periodization required is robust, and the mental training during the phases, will, as it has for thousands of others, release insights that have here to forth been lacking in depth and understanding. There are only a few coaches who have made major breakthroughs in training. Myself and my colloquies have touched on the mental aspects in ways few have imagined. For instance, when I worked with Esalen founder, Michael Murphy, his imagination sprang into action, and the combinations of meditating and running brought about new frontiers. We created the shesshin (mixed meditations) that have astounded groups providing and resulting in clarity and new distance abilities that they were able to express forthrightly after the training.

As much an art as a science, and infused with a glimmer of unique insight, the master coaches conceive the performances of their athletes as a personalized blend of insights and illuminated thinking that is unique to their personal insights. We can count these coaches who made unique contribution to only a few, and each was insightful in their own manner, and I will talk about some that influenced my life and coaching approach.

I have had the privilege of training under the finest running coaches in the history of middle-distance running. I have also melded it together with the most complimentary methodologies of the human potential movement of which, I can humbly say I am a pioneer. You can find this information in my website at spinorunning.com. The training you receive on the site has been gathered from my 60 years of coaching and includes what I have learned about mental focusing during my years as a teacher and as Director of the Esalen Sports Center within the world famous Esalen Institute.

Come look at my website spinorunning.com

I have put these trainings together in my website called spinorunning.com, and they have been time tested over decades and have proven extremely effective for all who utilize it. The two main programs for the recreational athlete have been repeated many times and are always on target to improve in the mile or 5k. It is presented with mental training exercises that fit into whichever phase of training you are using. For instance, in cross-country that moves into middle distance running, you will find your perfectly suited training under the categories of emerging, initiate, and the gold standard the program is for 12 weeks and goes through the segments (4) from conditioning to types of intervals and finishes with a few weeks in late May and early June when the runner is doing speed work and racing and persuadably reaching their best times of the year.

On the website spinorunning.com, through practice, you will discover how the mind and body integrate slowly into oneself. It will be slight changes but slowly you will notice them in your mind and body movements. These detailed workouts and mental training techniques go through progressive phases of from conditioning to multi-interval and classic interval training to speed workouts that allow one to reach peak functioning during the championship races of the season that matter most. During the championship races the combinations return to "full bloom."

Some of these ideas are presented in my six books including *Beyond Jogging: The innerspaces spaces of running* which can be purchased on Amazon and has been published in numerous languages, including Spanish, German and the latest, in Japanese, in 2021.

Let me explain some of the elements within the elite middle-distance running schedule you will receive by purchasing a personal program on spinorunning.com. A most significant contributor to my methods of running training is a Hungarian born master coach, Mihaly Igloi. He emigrated to the United States after escaping the Soviet takeover of his country in 1955. At that point, he had coached more under 4-minute milers with his method, than all of the other coaches combined. Numerous world record holders achieved success using his method that derived from research done by the legendary scientists Gerscher and Rendell, before the Second World War. The method is based on from the Freiberg interval system they developed. Basically, the running training is comprised of short intervals in sets with varying rest periods and allows for a whole team to train together at some time with even the slowest with the fastest for some amount of time. The pair of researchers noticed that short intervals at various speeds improved middle distance times. The most recent was Jim Beatty who ran the first indoor 4-minute mile. I trained in running and coaching with Master Igloi in 1966/67. I didn't run under 4 minutes; however, I learned his method. As I was the only college student, we would go to breakfast together, and he would explain his method with lots of X's and overlapping O's.

All runners' experiences this *Within Running Groups*

We all know that if your group runs together for a distance run, it will break up into various sections—fast ones in the front and others in various groups following. With this interval training, everyone can run at least some of the workout with their teammates. I have seen Igloi train four or five groups at the same time, mixing and matching them and finishing their workouts in the same amount of time. This adds to community, and everyone is helping or participating with each other.

Below was my experience with running and mysticism long before I had my mentor, Michael Murphy.

The inside story of the following narrative

The coach within this story of a mystical run was Jack Scott. An infamous rabble rouser, he had our group take over the track team at Syracuse University. Perhaps he is best remembered as the person who took Patti Hearst and protected her from police after the fire that killed her compatriots in the Symbionese Liberation Army one horrid night in LA. With his parents (former Irish republican army members) driving to their farm in Scranton, she was hid her out after she had been involved in various bank robberies, and thefts. It was part devilry. part humanitarianism, and what being around Jack he sometimes involved our group in merriment. The following is an example of such a time a time and has been published numerous times.

Running as a spritual experience.
MIKE SPINO, SPRING 1971

Weather is different every day; running has its shades of sunshine and rain. At Syracuse, I ran daily in the worst weather imaginable. Because of the hard winter, my running mate and I had an agreement that we would never talk while running. Snow covered many of the roads, so out of convenience, with only slight variation, we ran the same course almost every day. After classes, we would return to our rooms and prepare to run. To watch us get ready, you would have thought us looney. First, there was long underwear, shorts, and hood. Next, socks, for hands and feet, and Navy knit caps. The run was always better because you could think of a warm shower, and know that the nervous feeling, preceding the daily task of running, would be gone.

Eastern winters linger into spring, but one day the sun shone in a different way. Snow still curbing the road, but the inside pavement, where the black-brown dirt met cement, looked almost bounceable. Earlier in the day, the spirit of approaching spring made us, my coach, my running mate, and I, decide on a formidable venture. At a place beginning in the mountains and ending in a valley near the city, we had a six mile stretch which was part of a longer, twenty-mile course. We decided to run the six miles as fast as possible. The plan was for our coach to trail us with his car, and sound his horn as we passed each mile. Marty, my running mate, was to run the first three miles, jump in the car for the next two, and finish the last mile with me. We traveled to the starting point which was out of the sunshine, into the late afternoon mist. Our coach suggested a time schedule he thought we could run. I was sure I couldn't keep the pace; Marty said nothing, taking an "If you think you can do it I'll try, since I'm not running the whole way" attitude.

Almost even before we started, cars began to back up behind ourcoach's car, but he continued to drive directly behind us, and the cars soon tired of sounding horns and drove around all three of us. From my first step, I felt lighter and looser than ever before. My thin shirt clung to me, and I felt like a skeleton flying down a wind tunnel. My times at the mile and two miles were so fast that I almost felt I was cheating, or had taken some unfair advantage. It was like getting a new body that no one else had heard about. My mind was so crystal clear I could have held a conversation. The only sensation was the rhythm and the beat, all perfectly natural, and everything part of everything else. Marty told me later that he could feel the power I was radiating. He said I was frightening.

Marty jumped back into the car. There were three miles to go; it was still pure pleasure. A car darted from a side street; I had to decide how to react, and do it, both at the same time. I decided to outrun the car to the end of the intersection. The car skidded and almost hit our car, but, somehow, we got out of danger and had two miles to run. The end of the fourth and the start of the fifth mile was the beginningof crisis. My legs lost their bounce. I struggled to keep my arms low, so they wouldn't swing across my chest and cut off the free passage of air. My mind concentrated on only one thing, to keep the rhythm. If I could just flick my legs at the same cadence for a few more minutes, I would run a fast time.

Slowly, I realized I was getting loose again. I knew then I could run the last mile strongly. Perhaps, there is such a thing as second wind. Whatever, Marty jumped from the car when a mile remained, but after a few hundred yards he couldn't keep pace, so he jumped back in.

In the last half mile, something happened which may have occurred only one or two times before or since. Furiously I ran; time lost all semblance of meaning. Distance, time, and motion were all one. There were myself, the cement, a vague feeling of legs, and the coming dusk. I tore on. The coach had planned to sound the horn first when a quarter-mile remained, then again at the completion of the sixmiles. The first sound barely reached my consciousness. My running was a pouring feeling. The final horn sounded. I kept on running. I could have run and run. Perhaps I had experienced a physiological change, but whatever, it was magic. I came to the side of the road and gazed, with a sort of bewilderment, at my friend. I sat on the side of the road and cried tears of joy and sorrow. Joy at being alive; sorrow for a vague feeling of temporalness, and a knowledge of the impossibility of giving this experience to anyone.

We got back into the car and drove. Everyone knew something special, strange, and mystically wonderful had happened. At first no one spoke. Our coach reminded us that the time I had run was phenomenal compared to my previous times. At first, we thought the car's odometer might be incorrect, so we drove to a local track and measured a quarter mile. It measured correctly.

On the way home, I asked the coach if he would stop at a grass field, near our house. I wanted to savor the night air; I wanted to see if the feeling remained. It did, and it didn't. I have never understood what occurred that late afternoon; whether it was just a fine run, combined with the dusk, as winter was finally breaking, or finding out who and what I was, through a perfect expression of my own art form. It still remains a mystery.

WHY SOME COACHES ARE MASTERS

Master coaches have their own unique and often artistic style. They think outside the box and see running as more than just putting one foot in front of the other. For instance, the Australian coach Percy Wells Cerutty, was brought to Esalen in 1974 (I was the last person to receive a diploma from him). He focused on areas like breathing and surging and even experimented with runners cantering and galloping asymmetrically as a horse moves.

Just as early training is based on conditioning there are mental exercises that match each phase of training. Beginning with the full body recovery and sitting relaxation exercise, the training is formed "step by step" increasing mind and body connections in small increments. It may be as short as 20 to 30 seconds utilizing Soft Eyes™ that infiltrates the training. We explain the process on the website and use a post run technique called the Wipe Away™. The combination of these methods allows the runner to condense and mentally review the moments in and outside of the mental imaging and getting more used to both awareness's. You can use it, for instance, when tiring in practice or in a race to pull yourself to the next pole in a run, or to a location on the track. All of this is explained with videos on the website, spinorunning.com

Mind/body unity for a track runner takes a little time, and there are some transitions and experiences that are more basic than others. Recovering after the workout using a technique called "full body recovery" is one of these post workouts experiences. By focusing on post workout sensibilities using the technique derived from the work of Edmund Jacobsen, the inventor of Progressive Relaxation. By tightening and relaxing your muscles in various locations within your body, you can locate sore spots, notice them by tighting and relaxing them so you will gain knowledge of your body/mind for the next workouts. This exercise has shown to be very affective as a recovery technique.

As the last person to train with Master Coach, Percy Wells Cerutty, I was able to learn how he inspired his athletes. For instance, he would place statues around like thinkers and philosophers Goethe and Plato. Instead of having lap times within one's mind when racing, he prepared his runners to think more lofty ideas like 'the origins of the universe' and 'man's place on the planet'. Before a race he would motivate his runners by running himself to exhaustion as a tribute to their upcoming races. When his finest athlete, Herb Elliott, was winning the 1960 Summer Olympics for 1500 meters, Percy jumped over a security fence, took off his shirt and waved it to signify a world record was possible. He was taken off the edge of the track by a policeman.

The techniques in the programs of spinorunning.com have been researched many times to prove their effectiveness. They always work for both maximum enjoyment and improved performance, and there are reasons for these improvements. Firstly, the program is based on the idea of interval training. It is no coincidence that companies like Peloton, for instance, base their workouts on the interval (stop and go training) concept. This is derived from the concept of the Exercise Heart Range that a heartbeat is 220 minus your age, and 65-85% of that number will always improve fitness. We check these often in our training by applying gaits and tempos of running to our athletes. I tested this with a 12-year-old girl pedaling next to me on an indoor bicycle. She adhered to the 220-age and 65-85% output, and it was an interesting observation that I know would, if mixed correctly, add to her fitness.

Look on website for these programs:

* *Two Week Starter Program*
* *Treadmill for Recreational Program*
* *Program Chart*

THE COACH OF THE FUTURE

Recently, I wrote an article called, "The Athlete of the Future." If the ideas of that piece are relevant, then this essay about coaches intertwines. "The Coach of the Future," is intended to capture a glimpse of the types of people/coaches who have that magic something of elegance within them. It is hoped these teams and individuals will discover each other in the flow of ideas that match the aspirations of each. Together, right attitudes can take both the coach and athlete to a high level of compatibility. Perhaps sport may be the one vehicle that makes us more fit and better people when performed in this way.

Looking back—All our backgrounds have a similar tread!

Every person who has played youth sports remembers their most influential coach when they were growing up. He/She generated an idea to us of the possibilities of sport during our friendships. These significant coaches, even if only a few in your past, have great meaning for each athlete's journey. Significant situations are relative; we read about the championship coaches, and we have the community coaches that fill our lives. Each has a place in our development.

Cerutty, has said of leadership that "the way-shower" will emerge when the athlete is ready for him or her. People meet on purpose or by chance, and it is a process that has been happening ongoing in sport and civilization for generations. Anthropologist Margaret Mead has said that small groups of people make the greatest breakthroughs. While Sweden was neutral in WWII and Arne Anderson and Gunder Haegg, training under Gosta Holmer, almost broke the 4-minute mile missing by only one second.

The coach of the future will be imaginative

The image of the tough, whistle-around-the-neck, acting on fear and intimidation will be fading as more scientific coaches and psychologically-oriented coaches have the tools to instill confidence in their charges. Sixty years ago, when I was a championship athlete in a school that didn't have a cross-country team, a person emerged from the neighborhood and committed himself to my success. Often, like in this situation, I don't remember where we met or how the relation began; however, like Percy predicted, "the way-shower" does emerge when the athlete needs him or her.

I have been a running coach for almost 50 years and cherish the books and relations I have had in all those years of mentoring. I've coached world-class athletes and striving youngsters and learned something from all of them. What comes first to mind is the story of Joe Newton, who coached high school in Illinois and even Olympic Gold Medalist Sebastian Coe stayed with him during the '84 Olympics. He had over 100 young kids come out for cross-country each year, and he would give every one of them a nickname, which is something I have also done over the years. My best track friend says progress is when the athlete, as a runner, doesn't need the coach and knows enough to coach him or herself. I don't really agree with that and more wonder if there is a middle ground because it isn't just the workout or the game plan, but all the different aspects covered in this article. There is always more to teach and learn.

On the big stage there are coaches like Phil Jackson who take a Zen approach towards coaching. When coaching the competitive egos of star NBA basketball players, he would often not intervene in personal conflicts but observe and work through the relationships within the team. He would intervene indirectly by pinpointing who was trusted within the team among the players and often work through him to converge the team together.

The enthusiasm of football coach Pete Carrol is an inspiration. As the oldest coach in the NFL there is no one more enthusiastic. How does one maintain that level of fervor, loving the game and caring for each person on the team? Figuring out who gells with who is one of his gifts.

The wonderful coach at Canton College in Ohio became a close friend. At Life University, where I coached, when we got good, he didn't become bitter but rather helped in our transition to 12 national championships. We met me once at a conference and immediately knew my name.

So, in our modern age, what are the characteristics of the coach of the future? First, he/she will have the athlete's whole self as their main interest. Athletes may disappoint or be difficult, but the long-term welfare of each is the end goal.

We want to win, and will win, with the caring approach; however, sometimes the victory is from a different source. As a college coach, I won many national championships and have been elected to the Hall of Fames as athlete and coach, and the memories of the relations with the students who came back to see me on occasion are cherished.

In conclusion, it is not random luck (although in some situations it might be) why some runners improve and enjoy the running experience more than others. There is no better feeling to know that you are ready for a personal result and be able to pull it off. Both Peter Snell in *Drums* and Herb Elliot in *the Golden Mile* describe this feeling in their books. When you are in shape, it is a real enjoyment, and the yield of a time well spent in planning and preparation. I want this for the athletes I coach through my website.

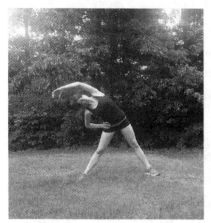

My daughter Marissa leading a stretch

My coach Percy Wells Cerutty-The Inimitable

Cerutty recognized not only for his world-record-breaking athletes, but for his free spirit, innovative methods and open imagination he imbued to all who met him at every level of fitness and health. I was the 20th and last person to receive a diploma to teach his techniques when he visited the United States for the Esalen Sports Center in 1974. Afterwards, I went to his training camp located in Portsea, Australia, a suburb of Melbourne.

His ultimate goal was not only to inspire but to liberate each person's free spirit by means of sport participation. He did this through creating a way of living he called, "Stotanism," that encompassed a lifestyle of robust individualism. Within, there were numerous aspects to his methodology. For instance, a running technique to improve stride by having the person run asymmetrically as a horse gallops and opening and closing of the hands during inhalation and exhalation as depicted on the cover of the Japanese translation of his book, *How to Become a Champion,* just published in Japanese by Mokusei Publishers

The book also describes the health benefits of strength through barbells and the charging up a sand dune, which he did with his athletes on his ocean-front training camp and timing distances within the schedules of his champions like Herb Elliott, as well as the tyros visiting on the occasional weekend. The book was written in the time frame of the 1964 Tokyo Olympics when he was uniquely honored for his contribution to innovations in sport practices.

Percy's dietary recipes mirror the latest trends in nutrition, as a self-proclaimed lactovegetarian. He was a transformationalist who created paradigms separate from all of today's running coaches. Other coached athletes may run fast; however, they don't seem to have the same open and expressive nature as do his runners or those whom he influenced to optimum fitness in one of his other six books called *Be Fit or Be Dammed*.

There are coaches who do take some parts of his training philosophy and apply it; however, very few possess his fiery personality, internal wisdom and ability to touch directly within the athlete to bring out the best for revamped and larger selves. There may never be another athletic coach who had a touchstone for the future as Percy Cerutty; his encouragements brought out the best in all of us.

I wanted to prove scientifically if my system worked and with the wonderful help of Bill Straub (a baseball catcher by trade who never asked a nickel from me for my mentoring), Mike Boit of Kenya, and Claude Sobrey. It all worked out for me to get my Ph.D., included as an appendix in this book.

How to Train and peak for cross-country and middle distance running. Get the full program for cross-country and elite distance running on Spinorunning.com

There are now millions of young people running cross-country and middle-distance races from 800 meters to 5,000 meters throughout the world. While it is a relatively easy task to put together a schedule of training for these events, there is little precise knowledge about how the most outstanding coaches in history approached the task. As much an art as a science and infused with a glimmer of unique insight the master coaches conceive the performances of their athletes as a personalized blend of insights and illuminated thinking that is unique to their personal insights. We can count these coaches who made unique contributions on a few hands and each was insightful in their own manner, and I will talk about a few that influenced my life and coaching approach.

In conclusion, it is not random luck (although in some situations it might be) why some runners improve and enjoy the running experience more than others. There is no better feeling to know that you are ready for a PR and be able to pull it off. When you are in shape for it is a real enjoyment and the yield of a time well spent in planning and preparation. I intend to become a frequent contributor to sportsedtv, and share my insights of 50 years of coaching and thinking about outcomes of mind and body within my books. Next time, I will be exploring the intracity of breathing and show where it is not just volitional but that there are techniques and methods to improve your breathing efficiency and functionality.

APPENDIX- DEMONSTRATING RESULTS

THE Performance of College Age Distance Runners

Michael P. Spino[1*], William F. Straub[2*]

1* Sports Administration, Kinesiology and Health,

Georgia State University, Atlanta, GA 30303

2*Department of Psychology, Tompkins Cortland
Community College, Dryden, NY 13053

2* wstraub7314@gmail.com

Abstract-**The purpose was to determine if Event Rehearsal Imagery (ERI) and Internal guided Imagery with Distractions (IGID) resulted in improvements in the running performance of college students. The participants (N = 74) were students at Kenyatta University in Nairobi, Kenya. Cooper's 12 min run test was used to assess running performance. Following 8-weeks of training, findings indicated that there was a statistically significant difference (0.05 level) in running performance between the Event Rehearsal Imagery (n = 29), Event Rehearsal Imagery with Distractions (n = 16) and the Control group (n = 29). Overall, there was a significant mean difference in running among male (n = 47) and female (n = 27 participants.**

Keywords- Kenya; Mental Training; Running; Cardiovascular Endurance

I. INTRODUCTION

Although Kenya is the running capital of the world, little attention has been given to the mental training of college age students. For the most part, the focus of mental training in Kenya and abroad has been on elite high school, college, Olympic and professional players. The truth of the matter is that mental training, which includes relaxation, concentration, imagery, goal setting, team building and cognitive restructuring, should be for everyone. According to Haversack [1], the health value of mental training has been clearly established. Her relaxation and visualization techniques have been used by persons who suffer from a wide variety of illnesses, including cancer, hypertension, anxiety, post-traumatic stress, depression and other illnesses. This investigation will add to the growing body of knowledge about the effects of distractions on running performance of college age students.

This review will cover two topics that are related to this investigation, i.e., the effect of mental training without distractions and the effect of mental training with distractions. First, we will present evidence for the effect of mental training (MT) on sport performance. Reviews of the literature on this topic were reported by: Richardson [2], and Feltz and Landers [3]. In another meta-analysis, Lander [4] answered a long-standing question in the sport psychology literature: Does a given amount of mental practice prior to performing a motor skill enhance one's subsequent performance? Of 60 investigations yielding 146 effect sizes, the overall average effect size was .48. Landers concluded that mentally practicing a motor skill influences performance somewhat better than no practice at all.

More recently, reviews of the literature were also completed by Driskell, Cooper and Moran, [5], Weinberg and Comer [6], and Behnke [7]. All of these investigators found support for the use of mental training. However, mental training must be practiced systematically over time to gain enhancement of performance in a wide variety of sports. Weinberg [8] identified two distinct motivations underlying the desire for an athlete to improve performance, they were, extrinsic rewards and intrinsic motivation. Weinberg [8], Martens [9] and Rushall [10] all suggest that athletes should be encouraged to improve performance from intrinsic rather than extrinsic motivation. Behncke [7] summarized well when he stated: "mental skills training relies on a methodology of self-mastery, generated through self-knowledge, to enhance the psychological state of the individual" (p. 2.).

Raglan [11] has proposed a Mental Health Model (MHM) that links performance in sport to psychopathology. He stated that there is an inverse relationship between sport performance and psychopathology, i.e., as mental health worsens or improves performance should fall or rise accordingly. According to Raglin, there is now considerable support for this view. Studies have shown that between 70 and 85% of successful and unsuccessful athletes can be identified using general psychological measures of personality structure and mood state.

After a thorough and exhaustive review of the research and conceptual literatures by Plessinger [12], she concluded that mental imagery should be combined with physical practice to produce the most favorable results. In addition, she stated that mental imagery not only improves specific motor skills but it also seems to enhance motivation, mental toughness and confidence. To summarize, following several carefully conducted investigations it seems clear that mental training when coupled with physical practice has the potential to enhance performance in a wide variety of sports.

There is growing research and popular interest in the role of distractions in the enhancement of cognitive and psychomotor tasks. Russell, et al. [13] compared a post-exercise mood enhancement program across common exercise distraction activities. These investigators examined whether exercise under conditions of distraction (television watching, reading) differed significantly from exercise control conditions. College students (N = 53) were randomly assigned to: exercise while reading, exercise while watching television or exercise control conditions. The POMS (Profile of Mood States Questionnaire) was used to assess pretest and posttest mood. Their findings indicate that it may be the enjoyable characteristics of distraction, and not distraction that are important in the exercise mood-enhancement relationship.

Other investigators, e. g., Spink [14] investigated the role of distractions in facilitating endurance performance. He randomly assigned individuals (N = 36) to one of three experimental groups: dissociation group, dissociation/analgesic group, and a control group. Measures of leg-holding times and subjective pain ratings were obtained twice, once before the treatment and once after the treatment. Results indicated that individuals in the dissociation/analgesic group performed significantly better on the posttest than individuals in the dissociation and control groups. De Bourdeadhuij, et al. [15] examined the effects of distractions on treadmill running time in severely obese children and adolescents (10 boys and 20 girls). Participants, ranging in age from 9 – 17 yrs., they resided in a treatment facility for 10 months. Participants performed a treadmill test until exhaustion in four different sessions. There were two sessions at the beginning and two sessions at the end of treatments. Treatments were counterbalanced, one with attentional distraction (music) and one without distraction. Obese youngsters ran significantly longer during distractions.

In a classic investigation, Pennebaker and Lightner [16] reported the results of two experiments with students. In a field experiment, they found that focusing attention on external stimuli while running led to faster running compared to the processing of internal stimuli while running. And in a treadmill study, participants were forced to process internal sensory information, such as their breathing rate, reported a large number of symptoms relative to participants who processed external sensory information (headphones with street noises) or no information (wearing headphones but hearing no sounds). They explained the beneficial effects of attentional distraction as contributing to a higher perception threshold for bodily information that normally inform participants to stop.

In a literature review covering the past 20 years, Masters and Ogles [17] confirmed that distractions have a positive effect on the motor performance of exercise and sports performance. More specifically, they reported that association relates to faster performance, dissociation relates to lower perceived exertion and possibly greater endurance. Further, they indicated that dissociation is not related to injury but association may be.

To summarize, the above investigations show that the use of distractions to enhance sport performance is worthy of further investigation. A reported above, some studies show positive gains while other do not. Further research is need to clarify the distraction performance relationship.

With the results of the above investigation in mind, the investigators decided to add to the growing body of knowledge about the effects of distractions on the running performance of Kenyatta University students (N = 74). It was hypothesized that students who experienced distractions while imaging running would perform significantly better than students who did not have distractions while imaging their running performance. In addition, because of super muscular strength, it is hypothesized that male students will out-perform female students in running performance.

II. METHOD

A. Participants

Prior to data collection, ethical approval for this study was obtained from the members of the Department of Exercise and Sport Science at Kenyatta University. A convenient sample of participants (N = 74), ranging in age from 18 – 26 years, were selected from university students who were studying at Kenyatta University, Nairobi, Kenya. Since Kenyatta is a National University, participants were from the various geographical regions within the country. Based on availability, male (n = 47) and female (n = 27) students were chosen from various populations within Kenyatta University. Recruiting procedures produced approximately 30 participants from the general population, 30 students who have not been exposed to the subject area from the College of Exercise, Recreation and Sport Science, and 30 students from other departments within Kenyatta University. Students were recruited from the second to fourth class term.

B. Materials

Cooper's 12 min walk run test was used to measure running performance. According to Cooper, the test has established validity and reliability. Generally, a correlation of

0.65 or better was found for runs of greater than 9 minutes. Plastic cones were placed at intervals of 100 m around a measured 400 m grass tract. Seiko stop watches (SO56-B, Seiko, Tokyo) with 100-time splits were used to time participants. Announcement of times were provided a 4 m, 8 m and 10 m intervals and when one minute was remaining. Laps and segments of laps were counted by trained research assistants to assess the distance run by each participant.

C. Procedure

A pretest/posttest design was used to assess the effects of mental training on the middle-distance running performance of Kenyatta University students (N = 74). According to Babbie [18], this classic controlled quasi experimental design is appropriate when investigators desire to test the effectiveness of independent variables on dependent variables. Experimental treatments (n = 3) were randomly assigned to groups (n = 3). Because of class scheduling conflicts, the participants (N = 74) were assigned to groups based on availability. Therefore, ANCOVA was used to adjust final posttest mean scores for between group differences in running performance that existed prior to the start of this experiment.

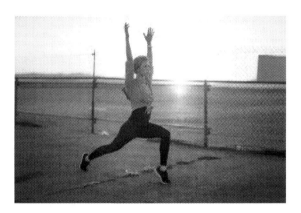

1) Pretest

Cooper's 12 min walk run test was used to assess running performance prior to the start of this investigation. Stop watches were used to time participants. It was explained to the groups that the intervals and specialized techniques were an antidote to constant one tempo running. Pacing strategies for increasing optimum energy while running has been defined as an issue by researchers using Cooper's test as an evaluative tool [24}). To accomplish the interval training pacing objectives, five different types of intervals were chosen to be run within and adjacent to the 400 m grass track. The researchers chose these interval distances because they represented a cross section of lengths that could be combined to achieve maximum physiological aerobic and anaerobic conditioning. They were: 80 m, 100 m, approximately 300 m, and two diagonals across the fields which were about 150 m. The complete length of the field, approximately 1000 m, was used to demonstrate the varied and increased pacing procedures used in the 24-Step Formula (Spino, [21].

2) *Experimental Treatments*

Following the initial assessment of running performance, each participant in the experimental groups received a 15 min. introductory lecture and explanation of the physical and mental training program. Internal, rather than external imagery, was chosen as the modality of chosen for this experiment. Gardner and Moore [19] suggest that internal imagery is more effective than external imagery.

The two experimental groups (Event Rehearsal Imagery and Event Rehearsal Imagery with Distractive Imagery) were taught the physiological principle of Exercise Heart Range which was used in their interval running training program. It was explained as follows: "The Exercise heart Range is a theoretical but practical construct based on a maximum heart rate of 220 bpm. The target for workouts that enable attainment of maximum fitness is to subtract a person's age from 220 and aim for 65 to 85 percent of this number" (Spino [20], p. 85).

A number of other techniques and concepts for enhancing pacing and assisting with mental concentration were taught to members of the experimental groups. They were fresh swing tempo, tidal breathing, soft eyes, surging, acceleration point, and 24 step formula.

It was explained to the groups that the intervals and specialized techniques were an antidote to constant one tempo running. Pacing strategies for increasing optimum energy while running has been defined as an issue by researchers using Cooper's test as an evaluative tool (Cooper, 1968). To accomplish the interval training pacing objectives, five different types of intervals were chosen to be run within and adjacent to the 400 m grass track. The researchers chose these interval distances because they represented a cross section of lengths that could be combined to achieve maximum physiological aerobic and anaerobic conditioning. They were: 80 m, 100 m, approximately 300 m, and two diagonals across the fields which were about 150 m. The complete length of the field, approximately 1000 m, was used to demonstrate the varied and increased pacing procedures used in the 24-Step Formula (Spino, [21].

3) *Training Methodology*

All experimental group members were taught the following techniques for improving the interval training, and strategic pacing. A five-point Likert scale was used to measure their effectiveness. The Control group did running at their own pace throughout the 8-wks experiment.

4) *Workout Techniques*

Workouts that are sections tied together with various segments are termed interval training. This means that the individual or group is moving at various intervals using a technique that corresponds to the desired cardiovascular workout. The following activities were used to train experimental group participants.

- *Fresh Swing Tempo* – A gait of running where participants move at about half speed, up to 50% effort. The purpose of the run is to increase the heart rate of participants at a low threshold of the Exercise Heart Range (HER).

- *Good Swing Tempo* – A gait of movement that enables participants to enter the middle and higher location of the HER.

- *Tidal Breath* – A technique of breathing that implements a full lung capacity enabling full acceleration into a faster gait of running.

- *Surging* – A technique of focusing while running by squeezing thumb to middle of first finger, making a 'ping' sound and accelerating into a faster tempo.

- *Acceleration Point Instruction* – The point at which a participant changes from one tempo to the next. To assist with this transition of pacing, participants used a surge or tidal breath.

- *Twenty-*Four Step *Formula* – A method of shifting pace (from light, to moderate to brisk) so that participants may utilize a wide variety of the EHR during each phase of the execution of each 24-steps.

5) *Experimental Groups Mental Training Techniques*

The following statements list and explain the techniques that were administered to members of the experimental groups. They enabled participants to integrate mental training techniques into their ongoing training program. At each venture, the goal was to be looking inward for a fresh perspective on the task ahead and to have an awareness of what is occurring within one's mind.

The objective of mental training was to introduce particular though patterns into the participant's mental outlook. The present study utilized a number of mind/body techniques. The 'Soft Eyes' technique was adopted form the martial arts and was used to enable participants to be able to 'look within' at the same time as safely running forward. "Stand and close your eyes- we will now practice a technique for looking inward. Close your eyes and imagine a large bird flying across the sky. Look at the feathers on his wings as he flies; notice the smoothness of his movements as he dips into a valley and then flies over the top of the mountains. Now open your eyes slightly, so that you can look out while at the same time viewing inward to your mind's eye to watch the bird in flight and view yourself with the same fluid motion as the bird. Now you will wipe the image from your mind by moving your fingers across your eyelids. By wiping your eyelids, you will be condensing the time that you are using 'soft eyes' and improve your ability to use the technique to your advantage when combining it with your running. By wiping the imagery away, you have established a beginning and end of this session. "Make a mental note of what has transpired in your mind and create a basis for your memory and remembrance" (Spino [21], p. 139).

6) *Guided Imagery with Distractions*

Distractive imaging was an intervention conducted during guided imagery rehearsal for participants (n = 19) in the Distractive Imagery Group (DI). Four times during the Event Rehearsal of the 12 min run, participants were distracted from the script and asked to roll over onto one side and find, and mark by crossing off a random number from a tally sheet. The object of this exercise was not to cross-off a correct number but the overall distraction it caused. Distraction research findings are equivocal (Bharani, Matthews & Sadhu, [22]. Some investigators contend that distraction may cause a decrement in performance; others believe that it can have a positive influence according to the type of stimulus (Bahrain, Matthew & Sadhu, [22]; Reisberg & O'Shaughnessy,

[23]. Distraction exercises may also be used to slow down peak performance or to stabilize a team that is out of union with each other.

7) *Post-test*

To determine the effect of experimental treatments on the dependent variable, Cooper's 12min walk/run test (Cooper, [24] was used to assess running performance. Plastic cones were placed at intervals of 100 m around a measured 400 m grass tract. Seiko stop watches (SO56-B, Seiko, Tokyo) with 100 time splits were used to time participants. Announcement of times were provided a 4 m, 8 m and 10 m intervals and when one minute was remaining. Laps and segments of laps were counted by trained research assistants to assess the distance run by each participant.

In addition to the evaluation of running performance, a questionnaire was used to determine the opinions of participants about the effectiveness of the training procedures. To determine the effect of mental training on running performance, the investigators' goal was to provide participants with a positive and satisfying mind/body experience while improving Max VO2 and running economy.

8) *Statistical Treatment of Data*

Analysis of Covariance (ANCOVA) was used to adjust final group mean distance running scores for initial mean differences that existed between the groups prior to the start of this experiment. A justification for using ANCOVA was to minimize the error variance associated with the use of class schedules rather than randomized groups. Data were collected at the beginning and at the end of this 8 – weeks experiment.

When significant F-ratios were found, Bonferroni's [25] procedures were used to locate between group differences. When using parametric statistical procedures, investigators should try and meet the basic assumptions of random sampling, normality, and homogeneity of variance. And, for multivariate experiments, there should be three times as many participants as variables (e.g., Keselman et al., [26].

Class scheduling prevented the investigators from fulfilling all of these basic assumptions. However, some statisticians (Box, [27]; Glass, et al. [28] have cogently stated that even if some of these assumptions are violated that these tests are rigorous enough to be used to analyze research data. From a contemporary perspective, Keselman, et al., [26] stated that "researchers rarely verify that validity assumptions are satisfied and they typically use analyses that are no-robust in assumptions to some degree" (p. 363).

Following tests for normality and homogeneity of variance of pretest and posttest scores, parametric statistical procedures were used to analyze the data. The Kolmogorov-Smirnov [29] procedures for normality indicated that pretest data were normally distributed among the three groups of participants. In addition, Levine's statistic for homogeneity of variance demonstrated that there was no significance difference (F (2, 71) = 8.46, p < .001) in the spread of scores away from their respective means among the three groups of athletes. Glass et al., [28] found that many parametric test are no seriously affected by violation of assumptions.

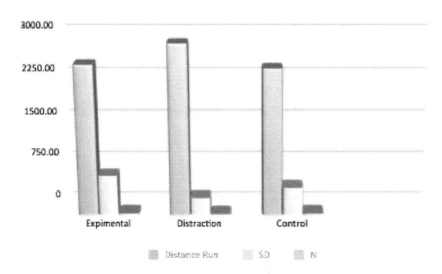

Having met the assumptions for normality and homogeneity of variance underlying the use of parametric statistical procedures, descriptive and inferential statistics were used to analyze the data. All hypotheses were evaluated at the 0.05 level of significance. When between groups statistical differences were found, Bonferroni's post hoc comparisons were made. Since random assignment of participants to groups was not possible, the three groups of participants (N = 74) were not equal in running performance following the pretest. Therefore, ANCOVA was used to adjust final posttest scores for initial differences in mean running performance that existed between the groups prior to the start of the experiment.

In addition, data analyses revealed that there were three outlier scores that exceeded 800 m. Therefore, the scores for Participants #40, #41 and #72 were eliminated from the analyses. Participant #1 did not take the posttest and therefore his data were also eliminated. The final sample sizes were: Experimental Group #1 (n = 29), Experimental Group #2 (n = 16), Control Group (n = 29).

III. RESULTS

The major null hypothesis H00 stated that there would be no significant between group mean differences in sport running performance, as measured by Cooper's Walk/Run test; In other words, this hypothesis stated that there would be no significant difference in mean running performance among Experimental Group #1 (n = 29) (ERGI), Experimental Group #2 (n = 16) (DI) and Control Group participants (n = 29) who did Event Rehearsal Guided Imagery (ERGI), Distractive Imagery (DI) and the Control Group (CG) activities.

Fig. 1 shows the mean posttest running scores and their stand deviations for the three groups of participants. Multivariate ANCOVA procedures (Table 1) indicate that his hypothesis was untenable. Wilks' Lambda = 0.91, $F_{(94, 132)}$ = 1.59, $p < 0.05$, $\eta 2$ = 0.045 showed that there were significant between group mean differences in running performance.

Fig.1. Posttest mean distance running scores (m)

TABLE 1 ANCOVA OF POSTTEST RUNNING SCORES
FOR GROUPS, GENDER, AND GROUPS BY GENDER
INTERACTION FOR KENYAN PARTICPANTS

Source	SS	DF	MS	F	p	η^2
Groups	527124.10	2	263562.05	* 3.02	0.056	0.83
Gender	913457.08	1	913457.08	* 10.45	0.002	0.14
Groups x Gender	239073.43	2	119536.72	1.37	0.262	0.04
Error	5854664.81	67	87383.06			
Total	5 26430000.0	74				

HO1 stated that there would be no significant difference in mean running performance among participants who participated in Distractive Imagery exercises (DI) and those who did Event Rehearsal Guided Imagery (ERGI). This hypothesis was accepted. Bonferroni's pair-wise comparisons indicated that there was no statistically significant mean difference between Experimental Group #1 participants who did (ERGI) and Experimental Group #2 participants who did DI. Although there was a 200meter mean difference between the two groups of guided imagery participants, this difference was not significant at the 0.05 level.

HO3 stated that there would be no significant difference in mean running performance between participants who did Distractive Imagery exercises (n = 19) and participants who were in the Control Group (CG) (n = 22). This hypothesis was accepted. Bonferroni's post-hoc test indicated that the 132.99 meter difference between these groups was not statistically significant at the 0.05 level.

HO4 stated that there would be no significant difference in mean running performance between participants who did Event Rehearsal Guided imagery and Control Group participants. This hypothesis was rejected. Bonferroni's post-hoc test produced a statistically significant difference between these two groups of participants. The mean posttest running performance of participants (n = 19) in the Distraction visualization group showed the greatest improvement form the mean posttest running scores of Control Group participants (n = 22). The direction of the improvement for participants (n = 19) in the distractive group was over 400 m, i.e., a lap further on a 400 m track.

Overall it is concluded that the experimental treatments were effective in enhancing running performance, i.e., from pretest to posttest the mean running performance of the three groups of participants improved. However, despite the fact that Experimental Group #2 (Event Rehearsal Distractive Imagery) participants had the highest posttest mean score, Bonferroni's post-hoc comparison did not produce a statistically significant difference from Control Group participants.

Table 2 shows the means, standard deviations and F-values for demographic, physical and mental training variables. Participants rated each training procedure on a five-point Likert type scale with a five indicating very effective and a one indicating that the training procedures were ineffective.

TABLE 2 UNIVARATE ANALYSIS OF DEMOGRAPHIC VARIBLES AND RESPONSES OF PARTICIPANTS ABOUT EFFECTIVENESS OF PHYSICAL TRAINING PROCEDURES

	Group							
	Experimental #1		Experimental #2		Control			
	(n = 39)		(n = 19)		(n = 22)			
Variable	M	SD	M	SD	M	SD	F	p
Age	22.26	1.04	22.37	1.77	22.86	1.83	1.23	0.31
Yr. Study	2.83	0.76	2.21	1.32	2.64	1.05	2.41	0.97
Birth Order	2.15	1.39	2.74	1.28	2.45	1.68	1.08	0.35
Surge	3.82	1.23	3.47	0.90	3.18	0.91	2.54	0.09
Fresh Swing	3.92	0.98	4.16	1.17	3.41	0.59	3.52	0.03
Good Swing	4.36	1.06	4.05	1.31	3.68	0.65	3.03	0.05
24-Step	3.72	0.99	3.05	1.47	3.86	0.99	3.07	0.05
Acceleration Point	3.82	1.02	4.05	0.97	3.55	0.74	1.51	0.23

df = 2 & 77

The training techniques were explained to the Control Group members to allow them to participate in the evaluation. As shown, statistically significant between groups differences were found for Surge, Fresh Swing, Good Swing and Twenty-Four Step training procedures.

For the Fresh Swing Variable, Bonferroni's post-hoc test indicated that significant differences were found between Experimental Group- #2 (DI) and Control Group participants. As expected, Experimental Group #2 (DI) participants (n = 19) found the Fresh Swing technique more effective than Control Group participants who did not actively participate in this training procedure.

For the Good Swing variable, Bonferroni's post-hoc procedures produced significant (0.05 level) between-group differences between Experimental Group #2 (DI) and Control group participants. In addition, a significant difference (0.05 level) was not found for the Good Swing variable between Experimental Group #1 and Control Group students.

Despite a significant F-value (F = 3.07, $p < 0.05$) for the Twenty-Four Step procedure, post-hoc between-group comparisons did not reach statistical significance at the 0.05 level. No other Bonferroni post-hoc comparisons reached statistical significance at the 0.05 level.

Overall, [Wilks' Lambda = 0.59, $F (20, 130) = 1.99$, $p < 0.05$, $\eta2 = 0.23$] indicated that there were significant between-group differences in the evaluation of physical and mental training procedures. In addition, there was a significant overall mean difference among male and female participants [Wilks' Lambda = 0.07, $F (10, 65) = 2.75$, $p < 0.01$, $\eta2 = 0.17$]. However, using Bonferroni's procedures, only one of the 10 variables reached statistical significance at the 0.05 level.

Gender Comparisons

Fig. 2 shows the mean posttest running scores for male and female participants. On the average, Male participants (n = 47) performed more effectively than Female participants (n = 27) on Cooper's Run/Walk Test. Males had a mean distance score of 2,770.09 m (SD = 56.71) while Females produced a mean yardage score of 2,343.64 m (SD = 110.27). The univariate ANOVA [$F (1, 67) = 10.24$, $\eta2 = 0.14$] was statistically significant at the 0.01 level.

Fig. 2 Running expectancy distances (m) for male and female participants

The assessment of the interaction of Gender x Group was also significant [Wilks' Lambda = 0.69, $F (10, 65) = 2.75$, $p < 0.01$, $\eta2 = 0.17$]. However, using Bonferroni's procedures, only one of the 10 variables reaches statistical significance at the 0.05 level. Males, on average, were older than female participants.

IV. DISCUSSION

The findings of the present investigation agree with the meta-analytic investigations of Feltz and Landers [3], Richardson [2], Weisberg and Comer [6], and Driskell, et al., [5]. All of these investigators found that mental training when coupled with physical practice enhanced sport performance.

These findings are also in agreement with the work of Hall and Erffmeyer [30]. They found that visuomotor behavior rehearsal when used with videotape modeling enhance the performance of intercollegiate female basketball players. In a classic study, Mahoney and Avenger [31] demonstrated that those gymnasts who did mental training made the US Olympic team more often than those athletes who did not do mental training. In summary, it is very clear that mental training when done well has the potential to enhance the performance of athletes in a wide variety of sports.

Since there are few investigations of the effects of mental training on ordinary students, it is unclear at this time of MTs contribution to the wellness. However, an important finding of the present investigation is that the participants really enjoyed and profited from the interventions that were used in this investigation. In support of the above finding, Mousavi and Mishkin [32] demonstrated that mental imagery reduced anxiety of tennis players, and improved their performance. The findings of the present investigation will add to the growing body of knowledge about MT's contribution to health and overall physical and psychological wellness.

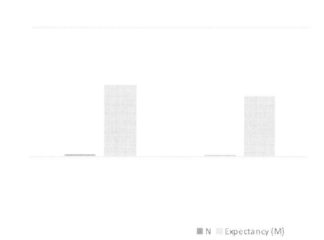

N   Expectancy (M)

Using college men and women as participants (N = 15), Straub [33] determined the effect of three different methods of MT on dart throwing performance. He found that Bennett and Pravitz [34], and Unestahl and Schill's, [35] procedures were effective in enhancing the dart throwing performance of these students. Despite receiving substantially less physical practice, students who practiced the MT of the above investigators significantly enhance their dart throwing performance.

Of course, a great deal more research is need to clarify the role of distractions in the enhancement of motor performance. For example, what types of distractions work best? How often distraction should be applied during the application of mental training procedures. Do skilled athletes, verses less skilled athletes, react differently to the use of distractions when attempting to enhance their performances? As often happens, research most always generates more questions than answers.

V. FUTURE RESEARCH

Despite extensive research during more than fifty years, there still remains many unanswered questions about the value of mental training and the effect of distractions on the performance of athletes. Although reviews of the literature by Feltz and Landers [3], Driskell [5], Weinberg and Comar [6], and more recently by Behncke [7] and Plessinger [11], show positive performance increments, some of these investigations they cite are lacking in experimental rigor. Using different experimental procedures and test that are sometimes lacking in validity, some of the above investigations are of little value. And although the use of meta-analysis is popular, some authorities indicate that it is like mixing apples and pears [36]. Walker, et al. indicated that meta-analysis is powerful but also controversial – controversial because several conditions are critical to a sound meta-analysis, and small violations of those conditions can lead to misleading results.

What is needed is to do investigations where experimental methods are careful monitored and treatments are extended over an entire season. The use of placebos groups are of course important and researchers need to use large sample sizes so that effect size is increased.

It is also unclear about what kind of distractions result in performance gains. In the present investigation a cross out sheet intervention was used to distract participants while they were visualizing their running performances. What would be a more viable procedure would be to audio and videotape distractions in the actual sport environment and see if these distractions affect sport performance. So to summarize, there is a dire need to carefully conducted investigations to determine the effect of distractions on the performances of athletes.

VI. ACKNOWLEDGEMENT

Appreciation is extended to the Kenyatta University students who participated in this investigation. Special thanks is extended to Kenyatta University research assistant Martin Yauma for his assistance in data collection. Thanks to supervisors: Dr. Michael Boit, Kenyatta University; Dr. Claude Sobry and Dr. Annie Mansy-Dannay, Lille2 University, Lille, France.

REFERENCES

[1] B-R. Naperscak, staying well with guided imagery. New York: Warner, 1995.

[2] A. Richardson. "Mental practice: a review and discussion," Research Quarterly, vol. 38, pp. 263-273, 1967.

[3] Feltz and D. Landers, "The effects of mental practice on motor skill learning and performance: a meta-analysis," Journal of Sport and Exercise Psychology, vol. 5, pp. 25-57, 1983.

[4] Landers, "The effect of mental practice on motor skill learning and performance: a meta-analysis." Journal of Sport Psychology, vol. 5, pp. 25-57, 1983.

[5] J. Driskell, et al.," Does mental practice enhance performance?" Journal of Applied Psychology, vol. 79, pp. 481-492, 1994.

[6] R. Weinberg and W. Comar "The effectiveness of psychological interventions on competitive sports," Sports Medicine, vol.18, pp. 406-418, 1994.

[7] L. Behncke, "Mental skills training for sports: a brief review," Athlete Insight, vol. 66, pp.1-18, 2014.

[8] R. Weinberg, "The relationship between extrinsic rewards and intrinsic motivation," in Psychological Foundations of Sport, J. Silva and R. Weinberg, Eds., Champaign, IL: Human Kinetics, pp. 177-187, 1984.

[9] R. Martens, Coaches guide to sport psychology. Champaign, IL: Human Kinetics, 1987.

[10] B. Rushall, Mental skills training for sports: a manual for athletes, coaches, and sport psychologists, Spring Valley, CA: Sport Science Associates.

[11] J. Raglan, "Psychological factors in sport performance: the mental health model revisited"., Sports Medicine, vol. 311, pp. 875-890, 2001.

[12] A. Pleasanter, "The effect of mental imagery on athletic performance." Nashville, TN: Vanderbilt University, Department of Psychology, 2007.

[13] W. Russell, et al., "A comparison of post-exercise mood enhancement across common exercise distraction activities." Journal of Sport Behaviour, vol. 26, pp. 368-383, 2003.

[14] K. Spink, "Facilitating endurance performance: the effects of cognitive strategies and analgesic suggestions," Sport Psychologist, vol 2, pp. 97-104, 1988.

[15] DeBourdeaudhuij, et al., "Effects of distraction on treadmill running time in severely obese children and adolescents," International Journal of Obesity, vol. 26, pp. 1023-1029, 2002.

[16] J. Pennebaker, et al., "Competition and internal and external information in an exercise setting, Journal of Personal Social Psychology, vol. 39, pp. 165-174, 1980.

[17] K. Masters, et al., "Sport psychology, "Associative and dissociative cognitive strategies in exercise and running 20 yrs. Later, what do we know?" Sport Psychology, vol. 12, pp. 253-270, 1998.

[18] W. Babbie, The basics of social research, Belmont, CA: Wadsworth, 2014.

[19] Gardner, et al., "A mindfulness-acceptance-commitment bases approach to athletic performance enhancement: theoretic considerations," Behavior Therapy, vol. 35, pp. 707-723, 2004.

[20] M. Spino, Beyond jogging: The innerspaces of running, Millbrae, CA: Celestial arts, 1976.

[21] M. Spino, Breakthrough: maximum sports training. New York: Pocket, 1985.

[22] S. Bharani, et al., "Effect of passive distraction on treadmill running using music," International Journal of Cardiology, vol. 97, pp. 305-306, 2004.

[23] D. Reisberg, et al., "Diverting subjects' concentration slows figural reversal, Perception, vol. 13, pp. 461-468, 1984.

[24] K. Cooper "A means of assessing maximal oxygen intake. Correlation between field and treadmill testing," Journal of the American Medical Association, vol. 203, pp. 201-204, 1968.

[25] C. Bonferroni, Elements of general statistics Italy: Florence: Seeber, 1930.

[26] Keselman, et al., "Statistical practices of educational researchers: an analysis of their anova, manova, and ancova analyses," Review of Educational Research, vol. 68, pp. 350-386, 1998.

[27] Box, "Non-normality and tests on variances," Biometrika, vol. 40, pp. 318-335, 1953.

[28] G. Glass, et al., "Consequences of failure to meet the assumptions underlying the fixedeffects analyses of variance and covariance," Review of educational Research, vol. 42, pp. 237-299, 1972.

[29] A. Kolomogorov – Smirnov. "On the determination of one empirical distribution of the Italian implement," Journal of the Gionrale Institute, vol. 4, pp. 83-91, 1935.

[30] E. Hall, et al., "The effect of visuomotor behavior rehearsal with videotaped modeling on free throw accuracy of intercollegiate female basketball players," vol. 5, pp. 343-346, 1983.

[31] M. Mahoney and M. Avener, "Psychology of the elite athlete: an exploratory study," Cognitive Therapy and Research, vol. 1, pp. 135-141, 1989.

[32] S. Mousavi, et al., "The effect of mental imagery upon the reduction of athletes' anxiety during sport performance," International Journal of Academic Research in Business and Social Sciences, vol. 1, pp. 342-345, 2011.

[33] W. Straub, "The effect of three different methods of mental training on dart throwing performance," the Sport Psychologist, vol. 3, pp. 133-141, 1989

[34] Bennett, et al., Profile of a winner: advanced mental training for athletes. New York, Lansing: Sport Science International, 1987.

[35] L-E. Unestahl and G. Shiller, Coaching with mental training, Sweden: Orebro: Schill Coaching AB, 2013.

[36] E. Walker, et al., "Meta-analysis: Its strengths and limitations" Cleveland Clinic Journal of Medicine, Vol. 25, pp. 431-439, 2008.

Michael P. Spino was born in New Jersey but has spent most of his adult years working in Atlanta, Georgia. He is an excellent track coach having coached at Georgia Tech and Life University. His teams have won many state and national championships. Recently he earned his doctoral degree at Lille2 University, Lille, France. Presently, he is teaching part-time at Georgia State University in Atlanta.

William F. Straub was born in Catskill, New York. He is a retired professor of kinesiology and sport psychology. He has published extensively in scholarly journals and now has a small private practice in sport psychology. He is a USOC certified sport psychology consultant. He received his PhD degree from the University of Wisconsin, Madison, WI and a Master's degree in clinical psychology from the new School for Social Research in NY

Printed in the United States
by Baker & Taylor Publisher Services